MASTERING YOUR FITNESS ROUTINE

A GUIDE TO USING THE WORKOUT APP ON THE

APPLE WATCH

AHMED .R

Contents

CHAPTER ONE

INTRODUCTION

With a built-in workout software that helps you track and get better at your exercise routine, the Apple Watch is more than just a gorgeous piece of jewelry. The Workout app offers a variety of features to support you in reaching your fitness objectives, staying inspired, and tracking your progress regardless of your level of experience as an athlete.

We'll look at how to track different kinds of workouts, examine your performance stats, and get the most out of your fitness regimens with the Workout app on the Apple Watch in this article. Setting objectives and personalizing workout metrics are just two of the many features that the Workout app provides to help you in your fitness pursuits.

The Apple Watch's Workout app is your go-to tool for monitoring, evaluating, and enhancing your workouts—whether you're riding a bike, running on the pavement, or doing strength training at the gym. Let's get started and learn how to get the most out of this effective exercise equipment.

An overview of the Apple Watch's workout app

The Apple Watch's Workout app is an adaptable tool that helps users track different kinds of physical activity, keep track of their fitness progress, and reach their wellness and health objectives. An outline of the main attributes and capabilities of the Workout app is provided below:

Activity Tracking: Users of the Workout app can keep track of a variety of physical activities, such as walking, swimming, cycling, rowing, and running. Users can select "Other" for activities not specified or from a selection of established workout kinds.

Personalization: Exercise configurations can be altered by users according to their tastes and fitness objectives. This includes customizing auditory cues and notifications during exercises, as well as setting goals for metrics like time, distance, calories burnt, and pace.

Real-Time stats: The Apple Watch shows real-time stats like heart rate, pace, distance, elapsed time, burned calories, and more when you're working out. It is simple for users to check their performance and progress by simply looking at their wrists while working out.

GPS Tracking: The Apple Watch uses its built-in GPS to track elevation changes, distance traveled, and route taken during outdoor activities like cycling, walking, and jogging. This lets users see their journeys on a map and gives them precise information about their outside workouts.

Heart Rate Tracking: During workouts, users' heart rates are continuously monitored by the Apple Watch's optical heart rate sensor. Together with other exercise parameters, this data is recorded and shown in real-time on the watch screen for examination at a later time.

exercise Summaries: Following an exercise, customers can see comprehensive performance summaries that include average heart rate, average speed, total distance traveled, and more. These summaries can assist users in identifying areas for improvement and offer insightful information about their fitness status.

Integration with Health App: The user's iPhone's Health app and the workout data stored on the Apple Watch are automatically synchronized.

This lets users see their past workouts, follow trends over time, and brag to friends and medical experts about their fitness accomplishments.

accolades and Awards: By giving users virtual accolades and awards for attaining milestones like finishing a particular number of exercises, scoring personal bests, or hitting activity objectives, the Workout app motivates users to stay active and motivated.

All things considered, the Apple Watch's Workout app is an effective tool for recording, observing, and enhancing physical activity. The Workout app gives users the resources and knowledge they need to stay inspired, stay active, and meet their fitness objectives regardless of their level of experience as athletes.

The Value of Fitness Tracking for Individual Health Objectives

Fitness tracking is essential for assisting people in reaching their own health objectives since it offers insightful information, motivation, and accountability. The following list of factors emphasizes the significance of fitness tracking for individual health objectives:

Accountability and Awareness: Fitness tracking brings attention to daily activity levels, workout routines, and general wellness. People can better understand their current fitness level and areas for improvement by tracking data like steps taken, calories burned, and activity time. To reach their objectives, people are encouraged to make better decisions and are held more accountable as a result of this understanding.

Setting Goals and Monitoring Your Progress: Fitness monitoring helps people to set quantifiable, targeted goals according to their health objectives, such as losing weight, strengthening their muscles, or improving their cardiovascular fitness. People may track their achievement, maintain motivation, and make necessary adjustments to their methods to stay on track towards their goals by routinely reviewing their progress and milestones.

Customization and Personalization: Exercise regimens and schedules may be made specifically for each person based on their preferences, fitness levels, and objectives thanks to fitness tracking. Whether it's jogging, cycling, weight training, or yoga, people may tailor their workouts to fit their interests when they have access to a wide range of exercise options. Personalized exercise regimens improve long-term outcomes by raising engagement and adherence.

Data-Driven Decision Making: By offering useful data insights, fitness tracking enables people to make well-informed choices regarding their fitness and overall health. People can pinpoint areas for development, maximize their training, and modify their lifestyle choices for improved health outcomes by looking at trends, patterns, and correlations in their activity data.

Motivation and Encouragement: Fitness tracking provides ongoing encouragement, incentives, and feedback to help people stay motivated and focused on their health objectives. Features that offer positive reinforcement and encouragement, such progress charts, achievement badges, and friendly competitions with friends or online groups, can motivate users to keep making healthy decisions by creating a sense of accomplishment.

Preventative Health Management: By spotting possible risk factors and early warning indicators, fitness tracking assists people in managing their health in a proactive manner. People can identify changes in their health state and take appropriate action, such as changing their exercise regimen, consulting a doctor, or changing their lifestyle to prevent future health difficulties, by tracking metrics like heart rate, stress levels, and sleep patterns.

Social Support and Community Engagement: A lot of fitness tracker apps have social elements that let users connect with friends, family, or other like-minded people for accountability, support, and encouragement. Participating in online communities, posting updates on one's progress, and taking part in virtual challenges all help to create a sense of community and camaraderie that enhances and prolongs the fitness journey.

For those aiming to reach their own health objectives, fitness tracking is a crucial tool.

Fitness tracking gives people the knowledge, control, personalization, responsibility, data-driven insights, motivation, preventative health management, and social support they need to take charge of their health, make healthy lifestyle choices, and eventually live happier, healthier lives.

How to Begin Using the Exercise App

The Apple Watch Workout app is easy to use and simple to get started with. Here's a quick tutorial to get you started tracking your fitness activities with the Workout app:

Using the Exercise App:

Find and press the Workout app icon on the main screen of your Apple Watch. Usually, it takes the form of a green icon with a moving figure.

Choosing a Type of Workout:

You'll see an array of available workout options when you launch the Workout app. To select the preferred training style, either scroll through the selection or utilize the Digital Crown.

Select the exercise program that best fits the activity you are going to perform by tapping on it. Common choices include cycling, elliptical training, rowing, outdoor walking, outdoor running, and indoor walking and running.

Choosing Objectives (Optional):

You might be able to set particular objectives for your exercise after deciding on a training style. These could be time, distance, calories burned, or other metric-based goals.

CHAPTER TWO

To modify your goals based on your tastes and fitness ambitions, use the "+" and "-" buttons.

Getting Started with the Exercise:

Press the Digital Crown or tap the "Start" button to start your workout after choosing your workout style and, if necessary, setting your goals.

Before the Workout app begins recording your activity, it will count down for a few seconds to give you a chance to get ready.

Keeping an Eye on Your Exercise:

The Apple Watch will show you pertinent real-time metrics for the exercise you've chosen while you work out. Metrics like elapsed time, distance traveled, pace, heart rate, calories burned, and more may be among them.

On the watch screen, swipe left or right to navigate between various metrics and displays.

Stopping or Resuming Your Exercise:

Press the "Pause" button on the watch screen to put your workout on hold. To continue, hit "Resume."

Press the watch screen firmly and then hit the "End" button to stop working out. Re-tapping "End Workout" will confirm.

Seeing the Workout Summary

The Apple Watch will show an activity summary, including total time, distance traveled, average pace, heart rate, and other pertinent stats, after your workout is over.

To get more information and metrics, scroll down. To get out of the summary screen, tap "Done".

Linking up with an iPhone:

The Health app on your associated iPhone will immediately transfer your workout data. To see your training history, trends, and in-depth insights, open the Health app.

Examining Exercises on an iPhone:

Open the Fitness or Activity app on your iPhone for a more thorough review of your workouts. View previous workouts, trends, accomplishments, and more right here.

Examining Enhanced Functionalities:

Explore more sophisticated features like heart rate zones, GPS tracking, specific exercise routines, and more as you get to know the exercise app to improve your fitness monitoring experience.

You may use the Workout app on your Apple Watch to track your workout activities and meet your wellness and health objectives by following these easy steps.

Establishing Your Preferences for Exercise

You may personalize your workout and improve the accuracy of your fitness activity tracking by configuring your workout preferences on the Workout app on your Apple Watch. Here's how to customize your fitness routine:

Getting to Your Workout Preferences:

Tapping the Workout symbol on the home screen will launch the Workout app on your Apple Watch.

Choosing a Type of Workout:

You can swipe up or down on the screen or use the Digital Crown to navigate through the list of possible workout options.

To adjust the workout type's preferences, tap on it. To change your options for outdoor running, for instance, choose "Outdoor Run".

Finding Exercise Options:

Press the watch screen firmly (Force Touch) after choosing a workout style to see more possibilities.

Select "Show All Metrics" to access training choices. You'll see options like "Set Goal," "Lock Screen," "End Workout Reminder," and so on.

Tailoring Exercise Preferences:

You can adjust a number of parameters in the exercise preferences section to suit your tastes. Typical choices include the following:

Metrics: Select the metrics you wish to view when working out. Elapsed time, distance, pace, heart rate, calories burned, and other variables are possible choices. To enable or disable each metric, flip the switches next to it.

Activate or deactivate haptic feedback (vibration) for certain messages, such as when you accomplish a new goal or are halfway through an exercise.

Set up alerts to tell you when you've completed a particular distance or time throughout your training. To suit your tastes, change the lengths and intervals.

Audio Cues: Set the pace, distance, duration, and other metrics' audio cues on and off. The audio cues' loudness and frequency can also be changed.

Enable screen lock to stop unintentional touches to the watch screen while working out.

journey tracking: To trace your journey and measure distance more precisely, turn on GPS route tracking if your exercise entails outdoor sports like cycling or jogging.

Preferences that are saved:

Press the Digital Crown or tap "Done" to return to the main exercise page after adjusting your workout choices.

For the exercise type you have chosen, your preferences will be stored and used for that type of activity in the future.

For Other Workout Types, Repeat:

If you prefer a different kind of training, follow the same procedures above to tailor each sort of activity.

You may personalize your fitness tracking experience to fit your unique needs and tastes by changing your workout preferences on the Workout app. This will help you stay motivated and reach your fitness objectives.

Commencing an Exercise Session

It's easy to get started with a workout with the Apple Watch's Workout app. This is how you do it:

Open the Exercise App:

Find and press the Workout app icon on the main screen of your Apple Watch. It appears to be a running figure on a green symbol.

Choosing a Type of Workout:

You'll find an array of potential workout types as soon as you launch the Workout app. To go through the list, either use the Digital Crown or swipe up and down on the screen.

Select the exercise program that best fits the activity you are going to perform by tapping on it. If you're going for an outside run, for instance, choose "Outdoor Run".

Choosing Objectives (Optional):

You might be able to set specific targets for your exercise, including time, distance, calories burnt, or pace, depending on the type of workout you chose.

To modify your goals based on your tastes and fitness ambitions, use the "+" and "-" buttons.

Getting Started with the Exercise:

You can start your workout by tapping the "Start" button or pressing the Digital Crown after choosing the preferred workout type and, if necessary, setting your goals.

Before it begins recording your activity, the Workout app will start a countdown timer, allowing you a few seconds to get ready.

Keeping an Eye on Your Exercise:

The Apple Watch will show you real-time metrics related to the chosen activity while you work out. Metrics like elapsed time, distance traveled, pace, heart rate, calories burned, and more may be among them.

On the watch screen, swipe left or right to navigate between various metrics and displays.

Stopping or Resuming Your Exercise:

Press the "Pause" button on the watch screen if you need to take a break from your workout for whatever reason. To continue, hit "Resume."

Press the watch screen firmly, then tap the "End" button to conclude your workout. Re-tapping "End Workout" will confirm.

Seeing the Workout Summary

The Apple Watch will show you an activity summary at the conclusion of your workout, which will include your total time, distance traveled, average pace, heart rate, and other pertinent data.

To get more information and metrics, scroll down. To get out of the summary screen, tap "Done".

Linking up with an iPhone:

The Health app on your associated iPhone will immediately transfer your workout data. To see your training history, trends, and in-depth insights, open the Health app.

With the help of the Workout app on your Apple Watch, you can quickly start a workout session and conveniently track your fitness activities by following these instructions.

Monitoring Your Exercise Outcomes

By utilizing the Workout app on your Apple Watch to track your workout progress, you can keep an eye on your performance, set objectives, and make well-informed decisions on your fitness regimen. Here's how to monitor your progress while exercise:

Getting to the Workout History:

On the iPhone you are partnered with, open the Fitness or Activity app.

To view your workout history, tap the "Workouts" option located at the bottom.

Seeing Performance Measures:

You can view a list of your most recent workouts arranged chronologically under the Workouts page.

To obtain comprehensive analytics and statistics about a particular workout, tap on it.

Examining the Workout Summary:

You may view an overview of important metrics like total time, distance, average speed, heart rate, calories burnt, and more in the detailed view of an exercise session.

If available, a map of your route, splits, heart rate zones, and elevation changes are displayed when you scroll down.

Examining Patterns and Perspectives:

Analyze patterns and insights from your workout data over time using the Fitness or Activity app.

Examine functions like monthly trends, weekly summaries, and accomplishments to get a better grasp of your performance and progress.

Creating Objectives and Obstacles:

Establish new objectives and challenges based on your past training experiences and performance indicators to push yourself further and reach new heights.

For extra encouragement, compete with friends and family using tools like Activity Sharing or sign up for community challenges.

Modifying Your Exercise Program:

Make adjustments and improvements to your fitness regimen using the knowledge you've obtained from tracking your workout success.

Decide which areas need work, such as stepping up the intensity, switching up the sorts of workouts, or concentrating on particular fitness objectives.

Keeping an eye on health metrics

During your workouts, pay attention to health indicators like heart rate to make sure you're exercising safely and within your target zones.

Analyze heart rate data patterns to determine your level of cardiovascular fitness and monitor your progress over time.

Honoring Successes:

Whether it's finishing a certain number of workouts, setting a new personal record, or accomplishing a particular objective, acknowledge and celebrate your accomplishments at each stage of your fitness journey.

To motivate yourself and encourage others, share your accomplishments on social media or with friends and family.

You may keep on top of your fitness goals, make wise workout decisions, and eventually get better outcomes by routinely documenting your workout progress and evaluating your performance indicators. When used in conjunction with the iPhone's Fitness or Activity app, the Workout app on your Apple Watch offers effective tools to support your fitness.

Stopping and Picking Up Exercises

Using the Workout app on your Apple Watch to pause and resume exercises is a handy tool that lets you take pauses during your activity without interfering with your tracking. This is how you stop exercising and start again:

Interrupting a Workout:

If you need to stop working out throughout your session:

To pause, just hit the "Pause" button on your Apple Watch's screen.

The timer will end and the Workout app will stop recording your activities.

If your Bluetooth headphones or earbuds are compatible, you may also interrupt your workout by pressing the "Pause" button on them.

Picking Up Where You Left Off:

To pick yourself back up after taking a break:

Press and hold the "Resume" button located on your Apple Watch's screen.

The timer will start up where you left off, and the Workout app will pick up where it left off in recording your movements.

As an alternative, you can continue your workout by pressing the play/pause button on the smartphone if you used Bluetooth headphones or earbuds to pause it.

Extra Advice:

Moreover, you can utilize Siri to pause and restart your workouts by uttering phrases like "Pause workout" or "Resume workout."

You can still store the data and examine your workout summary even if you unintentionally stop your workout rather than pause it.

When reviewing your post-exercise data, bear in mind that stopping your activity could have an impact on some indicators, including pace or heart rate.

You can take breaks during your activity without losing track of your progress by pausing and restarting workouts as necessary, guaranteeing a more realistic picture of your fitness session.

CHAPTER THREE

Stopping and Preserving Your Exercise

To guarantee that your activity data is recorded correctly, you must use the Workout app on your Apple Watch to end and save your workout. Here's how to wrap up and save your exercise:

Concluding Your Exercise:

When you're ready to complete an exercise during your workout:

To access the workout controls on your Apple Watch, press firmly on the screen.

Give the "End" button a tap. Usually, it's found in the screen's lower left corner.

As an alternative, you can use voice commands to finish your workout by saying "Hey Siri, end workout".

Preserving Your Exercise:

Your Apple Watch will ask you to confirm that you wish to finish your workout when you hit the "End" button.

To ensure that your workout has ended, tap "End Workout" one last time.

Seeing the Summary of Your Workout:

The Apple Watch will show a summary of your workout on the screen after you've finished.

Important parameters including total time, distance traveled, average pace, heart rate, calories expended, and more are included in this overview.

To see more information, including splits, heart rate zones, and elevation changes, scroll down.

Preserving the Data from Your Exercise:

To save your workout data, tap the "Done" button after viewing your workout summary.

Your exercise data will instantly sync with your associated iPhone's Health app.

Examining Your iPhone Workout:

To view and analyze your workout data in greater detail, use the Fitness or Activity app on your iPhone.

The app allows you to access your training history, analytics, trends, and accomplishments.

To see a more thorough summary of your fitness and health information, including workouts that your Apple Watch has logged, use the Health app.

You may be confident that your activity data is appropriately collected and can be utilized to monitor your fitness improvement over time by following these procedures to conclude and preserve your workout. You may use this information to set objectives, keep track of your progress, and make well-informed decisions regarding your workout regimen.

Examining Your Exercise Records

Understanding your performance, monitoring your progress, and making well-informed decisions about your fitness goals all depend on you analyzing the data from your workouts on your Apple Watch. Here's how to use your Apple Watch to evaluate your workout data directly:

Summary of the Workout:

Your Apple Watch will show a summary of your action on the screen after your workout is over.

Important parameters including total time, distance traveled, average pace, heart rate, calories expended, and more are included in this overview.

Specific Measures:

In the exercise summary, scroll down to see more information about your workout.

You may see stats like splits, heart rate zones, elevation changes, cadence (for running or cycling), and more depending on the sort of training.

Heart Rate Diagram:

You can see a graph of your heart rate variations during the exercise if your workout involved heart rate monitoring.

This graph shows you how your heart rate changed in relation to various workout intensities and stages.

Map for Exercises Outside:

When engaging in outdoor activities such as walking, cycling, or jogging, your Apple Watch may display a map of your journey right there.

Your GPS-tracked trip is shown on the map, so you can see where you traveled the greatest distance and visualize your route.

After-Workout Patterns:

Based on your most recent activities, your Apple Watch might offer trends or post-workout observations.

These insights could be in the form of warnings about notable accomplishments, recommendations for progress, or comparisons to earlier exercises.

Heart Rate Comeback:

A few workout reports might also provide details on how your heart rate recovered from the exercise.

After exercise, heart rate recovery the speed at which your heart rate returns to normal can serve as a gauge of your cardiovascular fitness.

Data Exchange and Export:

You can export your workout data for additional analysis or share it with others right from your Apple Watch.

Use your watch's sharing features to forward exercise summaries to loved ones, personal trainers, or friends.

Without requiring access to other devices or apps, you may obtain important insights into your performance, effort, and growth by evaluating your workout data immediately on your Apple Watch. You can use these insights to improve your training, make more reasonable goals, and maintain motivation as you pursue fitness.

Using Workouts and Advanced Features

You can improve your fitness tracking experience and more successfully meet your wellness and health objectives by making use of the sophisticated features and workouts on your Apple Watch. How to maximize these features is as follows:

Tailoring Exercise Measures:

Put the information that matters most to you front and center in the metrics that are shown to you during your workouts.

Open the Workout app on your Apple Watch, choose a workout style, and then adjust the metrics displayed while working out using Force Touch.

Establishing Alerts and Goals:

For your workouts, set specific objectives like time, distance, or calorie burn.

Turn on alerts to receive notifications when you complete intervals or reach milestones while working out.

HIIT, or high-intensity interval training:

Utilize the HIIT workouts that your Apple Watch offers to enhance cardiovascular fitness and burn calories to the fullest.

Choose from pre-planned HIIT exercises or design your own intervals based on your fitness objectives and degree of fitness.

Features of Outdoor Runs and Walks:

Get real-time pace and distance updates by utilizing GPS to track your routes while completing the Outdoor Walk and Outdoor Run programs.

Explore tools like Pace Alerts and Rolling Mile to keep on track and monitor your performance.

Swimming Workouts:

If you're a swimmer, employ the Apple Watch's waterproof construction and swimming workout mode to measure your laps, strokes, and distance in the pool.

Enable "Pool Swim" mode to precisely capture your swim parameters, including stroke type and pace.

Strength Training and Gym Workouts:

Track your strength training sessions and gym workouts by selecting the "Strength Training" or "Other" workout options on your Apple Watch.

Manually add details such as sets, reps, and weights lifted to keep a record of your strength growth.

Yoga and Mindfulness:

Incorporate yoga and mindfulness techniques into your routine using the Yoga and Mindfulness workouts available on your Apple Watch.

Follow guided sessions to improve flexibility, reduce tension, and boost general well-being.

Elevation Gain Tracking:

Monitor elevation gain and fluctuations in height during outdoor activities like hiking, trail running, or cycling.

Examine the data and elevation graphs in your workout summaries to determine how challenging your routes are.

Measurements of Heart Rate Variability (HRV):

To determine when your body is ready for activity and has recovered from an injury, monitor your heart rate variability (HRV).

To maximize recuperation and performance during your workouts, use the Breathe app or HRV assessments.

Connectivity with Outside Applications:

Use appropriate third-party fitness applications and platforms on your Apple Watch to get access to more training possibilities, analytical tools, and workout options.

You may customize your fitness regimen to your unique goals, interests, and activities by using the sophisticated features and workouts on your Apple Watch. This will keep you motivated and help you reach your fitness objectives more successfully.

Fixing Frequently Occurring Problems with the Exercise App

Although the Apple Watch's Workout app is generally dependable, you could occasionally run into problems that ruin your monitoring experience. The following are some typical issues and solutions:

Exercise Does Not Begin:

Make sure your iPhone and Apple Watch are correctly synced and have enough battery life if you're having trouble starting an exercise.

To restart your Apple Watch, press and hold the side button until the Power Off slider appears. Then, drag the slider to turn off the device. Then, to restart the Apple logo, tap and hold the side button once more.

Look for available software updates for your iPhone and Apple Watch. These updates can contain bug fixes that remedy problems with the Workout app.

GPS tracking or distance that is inaccurate:

If you experience inaccurate GPS tracking or distance during your outdoor workouts, make sure Location Services are turned on on both your iPhone and Apple Watch.

For your Apple Watch to receive a strong GPS signal, make sure it is facing the sky. Steer clear of obstructions that could impede GPS reception, such as towering buildings and dense trees.

Try using a few outdoor workouts with precise distance measurements and reliable routes to calibrate the GPS on your Apple Watch.

Problems with Heart Rate Monitoring:

Make sure the Apple Watch is securely fastened to your wrist and in the proper position if it isn't detecting your heart rate during exercise.

To avoid clogging heart rate sensors with debris, sweat, or dirt, clean the back of your Apple Watch and your skin.

To reset heart rate tracking features and fix any transient software issues, restart your Apple Watch.

Data from Workouts Not Syncing:

Make sure your iPhone and Apple Watch are in close proximity to one another and linked to the same Wi-Fi network if your workout data isn't synchronizing between them.

Make sure that your iPhone and Apple Watch have Bluetooth turned on, as this is how workout data is synced.

Make sure that the Workout app's ability to share workout data is enabled by opening the Health app on your iPhone and selecting the "Health Data" option.

Depletion of Battery During Exercise:

If your Apple Watch is draining its battery too much when you're working out, you might want to disable features that use a lot of power, such as Always-On Display and background app update.

To maximize battery life during exercises, adjust settings like screen brightness, haptic feedback, and audio notifications.

Restart your Apple Watch and think about contacting Apple Support for more help if the battery drain continues.

CHAPTER FOUR

Try troubleshooting the Workout app on your Apple Watch if the problem persists after trying several solutions. Apple Support can offer you individualized support and advice based on your unique circumstances.

Considerations for Security and Privacy

It's important to think about privacy and security when using your Apple Watch for exercise in order to safeguard your personal information and keep your mind at ease. The following are some crucial security and privacy factors:

Privacy of Location Data:

Your Apple Watch detects your location when you use GPS-enabled workouts, such outdoor cycling or running, to deliver precise distance and route information.

Share this location information carefully, particularly if you're posting routes or exercise summaries on social media.

To manage how your location information is shared with apps and services, check and modify your location sharing preferences in the Privacy settings on your iPhone and Apple Watch.

Protection of Health and Fitness Data:

During exercise, your Apple Watch records a variety of health and fitness metrics, such as heart rate, amount of activity, and type of workout.

To stop unauthorized access to your health data, make sure your Apple Watch is safely locked with a passcode or biometric verification (such as Face ID or Touch ID).

To have your Apple Watch automatically lock when not on your wrist, turn on the "Wrist Detection" feature.

Sharing and Syncing Preferences:

To manage the way your exercise data is shared across your iPhone, Apple Watch, and other devices, check your sharing and syncing preferences.

If you would rather keep your fitness data private, you might want to disable automated workout data sharing with other apps and services.

App Privacy Settings:

When allowing third-party fitness apps to interact with your Apple Watch, exercise caution.

Make sure these apps' data handling procedures and privacy policies match your privacy preferences by reviewing them.

Make sure you periodically check and remove permissions from applications that don't need access to your fitness and health information.

Data Security and Encryption Procedures:

Apple protects the health and fitness information on your iPhone and Apple Watch using strong encryption and security protocols.

Make sure the software upgrades on your devices are up to date in order to take advantage of security patches and improvements.

SOS Emergency Feature:

Learn how to use your Apple Watch's Emergency SOS feature, which enables you to promptly contact emergency services and alert your emergency contacts in the event of an emergency while working out.

Using the Apple Watch app on your iPhone, you can set up your SOS settings and emergency contacts.

You may reap the benefits of fitness monitoring while protecting your personal information and upholding your privacy settings by being aware of privacy and security considerations when using your Apple Watch for exercise. Make sure your privacy settings are in line with your needs and comfort level by reviewing and adjusting them on a regular basis.

To sum up, if you know how to use the Workout app on your Apple Watch, you can track and enhance your fitness journey in a whole new way. You may track your progress, get insights into your workouts, and maintain motivation to reach your wellness and health objectives by making the most of its capabilities.

We've gone over all the basics of using the Workout app in this guide, including how to start and stop workouts, adjust preferences, and view data. We've looked at cutting-edge features like heart rate monitoring, outdoor tracking, and HIIT workouts, which give you the ability to customize your exercise regimen to suit your requirements and tastes.

It's critical to keep in mind that perseverance and commitment are necessary for success. The Workout app on your Apple Watch is a dependable friend that will help you stay accountable and motivated at every stage of your fitness journey, regardless of your experience level.

Take advantage of the Workout app to challenge yourself, try new things, and create difficult objectives as you go. Along with developing physical strength, each workout also helps you develop resilience, self-control, and a better awareness of your body and its potential.

Put on your Apple Watch, lace on your sneakers, and use the Workout app as a roadmap to a more active, healthy lifestyle. Your Apple Watch is there to help you every step of the way, whether you're running on the pavement, working out at the gym, or hiking through the trails. Cheers to many more satisfying workouts and accomplishments on your path to fitness!

THE END

www.ingramcontent.com/pod-product-compliance
Lightning Source LLC
Chambersburg PA
CBHW051916250726
48659CB00002B/683